My Daily Keto Chame Breakfast Recipe Book

Easy and Healthy Recipes to Make Unforgettable First Courses

Kade Harrison

Table of Contents

Mozzarellas & Psyllium Husk Chaffles

Servings: 2
Cooking Time:
8 Minutes

Ingredients:

- ½ cup Mozzarella cheese, shredded
- 1 large organic egg, beaten
- 2 tablespoons blanched almond flour
- ½ teaspoon Psyllium husk powder
- ¼ teaspoon organic baking powder

Directions:

1. Preheat a mini waffle iron and then grease it.
2. In a bowl, place all the ingredients and beat until well combined.
3. Place half of the mixture into preheated waffle iron and cook for about 4 minutes or until golden brown.
4. Repeat with the remaining mixture.
5. Serve warm.

Nutrition:

Calories: 101 Net Carb: 1 Fat: 7.1g Saturated Fat: 1.8g Carbohydrates: 2.9g Dietary Fiber: 1.3g Sugar: 0.2g Protein: 6.7g

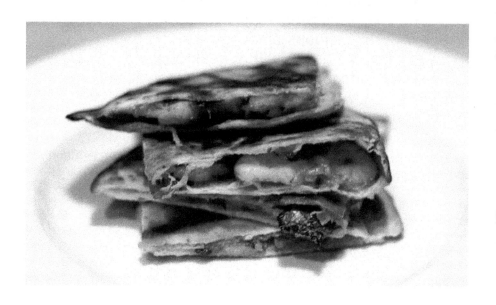

Pumpkin-cinnamon Churro Sticks

Servings: 2

Cooking Time:

14 Minutes

Ingredients:

- 3 tbsp coconut flour
- ¼ cup pumpkin puree
- 1 egg, beaten
- ½ cup finely grated mozzarella cheese
- 2 tbsp sugar-free maple syrup + more for serving
- 1 tsp baking powder
- 1 tsp vanilla extract
- ½ tsp pumpkin spice seasoning
- 1/8 tsp salt
- 1 tbsp cinnamon powder

Directions:

1. Preheat the waffle iron.
2. Mix all the ingredients in a medium bowl until well combined.
3. Open the iron and add half of the mixture. Close and cook until golden brown and crispy, 7 minutes.
4. Remove the chaffle onto a plate and make 1 more with the remaining batter.
5. Cut each chaffle into sticks, drizzle the top with more maple syrup and serve after.

Nutrition:

Calories 219 Fats 9.72 g Carbs 8.g Net Carbs 4.34 g
Protein 25.27g

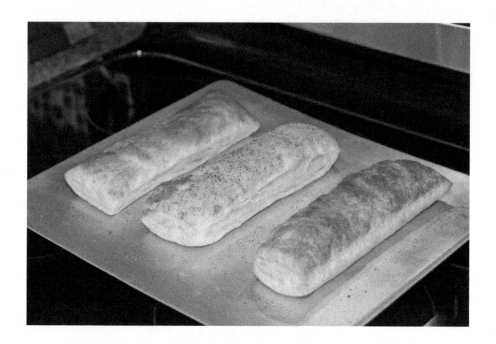

Chicken Jalapeño Chaffles

Servings: 2

Cooking Time:

14 Minutes

Ingredients:

- 1/8 cup finely grated Parmesan cheese
- ¼ cup finely grated cheddar cheese
- 1 egg, beaten
- ½ cup cooked chicken breasts, diced
- 1 small jalapeño pepper, deseeded and minced
- 1/8 tsp garlic powder
- 1/8 tsp onion powder
- 1 tsp cream cheese, softened

Directions:

1. Preheat the waffle iron.
2. In a medium bowl, mix all the ingredients until adequately combined.
3. Open the iron and add half of the mixture. Close and cook until crispy, 7 minutes.
4. Transfer the chaffle to a plate and make a second chaffle in the same manner.
5. Allow cooling and serve afterward.

Nutrition:

Calories: 201 Fats: 11.49g Carbs: 3.7 Net Carbs: 3.36g Protein: 20.11g

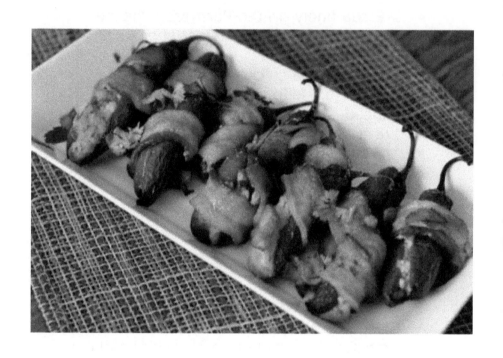

Chocolate & Almond Chaffle

Servings: 3

Cooking Time:

12 Minutes

Ingredients:

- 1 egg
- ¼ cup mozzarella cheese, shredded
- 1 oz. cream cheese
- 2 teaspoons sweetener
- 1 teaspoon vanilla
- 2 tablespoons cocoa powder
- 1 teaspoon baking powder
- 2 tablespoons almonds, chopped
- 4 tablespoons almond flour

Directions:

1. Blend all the ingredients in a bowl while the waffle maker is preheating.
2. Pour some of the mixture into the waffle maker.
3. Close and cook for 4 minutes.
4. Transfer the chaffle to a plate. Let cool for 2 minutes.
5. Repeat steps using the remaining mixture.

Nutrition:

Calories: 1 Total Fat: 13.1g Saturated Fat: 5g
Cholesterol: 99mg Sodium: 99mg Potassium: 481mg

Total Carbohydrate: 9.1g Dietary Fiber: 3.8g Protein 7.8g Total Sugars: 0.8g

Keto Chocolate Fudge Chaffle

Servings: 2

Cooking Time:

14 Minutes

Ingredients:

- 1 egg, beaten
- ¼ cup finely grated Gruyere cheese
- 2 tbsp unsweetened cocoa powder
- ¼ tsp baking powder
- ¼ tsp vanilla extract
- 2 tbsp erythritol
- 1 tsp almond flour
- 1 tsp heavy whipping cream
- A pinch of salt

Directions:

1. Preheat the waffle iron.
2. Add all the ingredients to a medium bowl and mix well.
3. Open the iron and add half of the mixture. Close and cook until golden brown and crispy, 7 minutes.
4. Remove the chaffle onto a plate and make another with the remaining batter.
5. Cut each chaffle into wedges and serve after.

Nutrition:

Calories 173 Fats 13.08g Carbs 3.98g Net Carbs 2.28g Protein 12.27g

Broccoli & Cheese Chaffle

Servings: 2

Cooking Time:

8 Minutes

Ingredients:

- ¼ cup broccoli florets
- 1 egg, beaten
- 1 tablespoon almond flour
- ¼ teaspoon garlic powder
- ½ cup cheddar cheese

Directions:

1. Preheat your waffle maker.
2. Add the broccoli to the food processor.
3. Pulse until chopped.
4. Add to a bowl.
5. Stir in the egg and the rest of the ingredients.
6. Mix well.
7. Pour half of the batter to the waffle maker.
8. Cover and cook for 4 minutes.
9. Repeat procedure to make the next chaffle.

Nutrition:

Calories 170 Total Fat 13 g Saturated Fat 7 g
Cholesterol 112 mg Sodium 211 mg Potassium 94 mg
Total Carbohydrate 2 g Dietary Fiber 1 g Protein 11 g
Total Sugars 1 g

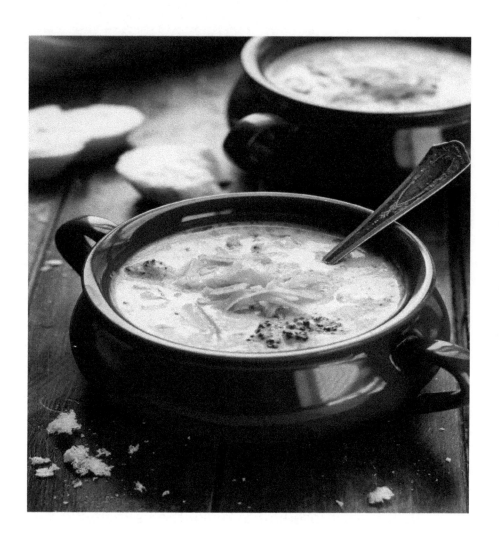

Chaffled Brownie Sundae

Servings: 4

Cooking Time:

30 Minutes

Ingredients:

- For the chaffles:
- 2 eggs, beaten
- 1 tbsp unsweetened cocoa powder
- 1 tbsp erythritol
- 1 cup finely grated mozzarella cheese
- For the topping:
- 3 tbsp unsweetened chocolate, chopped
- 3 tbsp unsalted butter
- ½ cup swerve sugar
- Low-carb ice cream for topping
- 1 cup whipped cream for topping
- 3 tbsp sugar-free caramel sauce

Directions:

1. For the chaffles:
2. Preheat the waffle iron.
3. Meanwhile, in a medium bowl, mix all the ingredients for the chaffles.
4. Open the iron, pour in a quarter of the mixture, cover, and cook until crispy, 7 minutes.
5. Remove the chaffle onto a plate and make 3 more with the remaining batter.
6. Plate and set aside.
7. For the topping:

8. Meanwhile, melt the chocolate and butter in a medium saucepan with occasional stirring, 2 minutes.
9. To Servings:
10.   Divide the chaffles into wedges and top with the ice cream, whipped cream, and swirl the chocolate sauce and caramel sauce on top.
11.   Serve immediately.

Nutrition:

Calories 165 Fats 11.39 g Carbs 3.81 g Net Carbs 2.91 g Protein 79 g

Cream Cheese Chaffle

Servings: 2

Cooking Time:

8 Minutes

Ingredients:

- 1 egg, beaten
- 1 oz. cream cheese
- ½ teaspoon vanilla
- 4 teaspoons sweetener
- ¼ teaspoon baking powder
- Cream cheese

Directions:

1. Preheat your waffle maker.
2. Add all the ingredients in a bowl.
3. Mix well.
4. Pour half of the batter into the waffle maker.
5. Seal the device.
6. Cook for 4 minutes.
7. Remove the chaffle from the waffle maker.
8. Make the second one using the same steps.
9. Spread remaining cream cheese on top before serving.

Nutrition:

Calories 169 Total Fat 14.3g Saturated Fat 7.6g Cholesterol 195mg Sodium 147mg Potassium 222mgTotal Carbohydrate 4g Dietary Fiber 4g Protein 7.7g Total Sugars 0.7g

Garlic Chaffles

Servings:4

Cooking Time:

5 Minutes

Ingredients:

- 1/2 cup mozzarella cheese, shredded
- 1/3 cup cheddar cheese
- 1 large egg
- ½ tbsp. garlic powder
- 1/2 tsp Italian seasoning
- 1/4 tsp baking powder

Directions:

1. Switch on your waffle maker and lightly grease your waffle maker with a brush.
2. Beat the egg with garlic powder, Italian seasoning and baking powder in a small mixing bowl.
3. Add mozzarella cheese and cheddar cheese tothe egg mixture and mix well.
4. Pour half of the chaffles batter into the middle of your waffle iron and close the lid.
5. Cook chaffles for about 2-3 minutesutes until crispy.
6. Once cooked, remove chaffles from the maker.
7. Sprinkle garlic powder on top and enjoy!

Nutrition:

Protein: 32% 36 kcal Fat: 61% 69 kcal Carbohydrates: 7% 7 kcal

Cinnamon Powder Chaffles

Servings:2

Cooking Time:

5 Minutes

Ingredients:

- 1 large egg
- 3/4 cup cheddar cheese, shredded
- 2 tbsps. coconut flour
- 1/2 tbsps. coconut oil melted
- 1 tsp. stevia
- 1/2 tsp cinnamon powder
- 1/2 tsp vanilla extract
- 1/2 tsp psyllium husk powder
- 1/4 tsp baking powder

Directions:

1. Switch on your waffle maker.
2. Grease your waffle maker with cooking spray and heat up on medium heat.
3. In a mixing bowl, beat egg with coconut flour, oil, stevia, cinnamon powder, vanilla, husk powder, and baking powder.
4. Once the egg is beaten well, add in cheese and mix again.
5. Pour half of the waffle batter into the middle of your waffle iron and close the lid.
6. Cook chaffles for about 2-3 minutesutes until crispy.
7. Once chaffles are cooked, carefully remove them from the maker.
8. Serve with keto hot chocolate and enjoy!

Nutrition:

Protein: 25% 62 kcal Fat: 72% 175 kcal Carbohydrates: 3% 7 kcal

Chaffles With Raspberry Syrup

Servings: 4

Cooking Time:

38 Minutes

Ingredients:

- For the chaffles:
- 1 egg, beaten
- ½ cup finely shredded cheddar cheese
- 1 tsp almond flour
- 1 tsp sour cream
- For the raspberry syrup:
- 1 cup fresh raspberries
- ¼ cup swerve sugar
- ¼ cup water
- 1 tsp vanilla extract

Directions:

1. For the chaffles:
2. Preheat the waffle iron.
3. Meanwhile, in a medium bowl, mix the egg, cheddar cheese, almond flour, and sour cream.
4. Open the iron, pour in half of the mixture, cover, and cook until crispy, 7 minutes.
5. Remove the chaffle onto a plate and make another with the remaining batter.
6. For the raspberry syrup:
7. Meanwhile, add the raspberries, swerve sugar, water, and vanilla extract to a medium pot. Set over low heat and cook until the raspberries soften and sugar becomes syrupy.

Occasionally stir while mashing the raspberries as you go.

8. Turn the heat off when your desired consistency is achieved and set aside to cool.
9. Drizzle some syrup on the chaffles and enjoy when ready.

Nutrition:

Calories 105 Fats 7.11 g Carbs 4.31 g Net Carbs 2.21 g Protein 5.83 g

Egg-free Coconut Flour Chaffles

Servings: 2

Cooking Time:

10 Minutes

Ingredients:

- 1 tablespoon flaxseed meal
- 2½ tablespoons water
- ¼ cup Mozzarella cheese, shredded
- 1 tablespoon cream cheese, softened
- 2 tablespoons coconut flour

Directions:

1. Preheat a waffle iron and then grease it.
2. In a bowl, place the flaxseed meal and water and mix well.
3. Set aside for about 5 minutes or until thickened.
4. In the bowl of flaxseed mixture, add the remaining ingredients and mix until well combined.
5. Place half of the mixture into preheated waffle iron and cook for about 3-minutes or until golden brown.
6. Repeat with the remaining mixture.
7. Serve warm.

Nutrition:

Calories: 76 Net Carb: 2.3g Fat: 4.2g Saturated Fat: 2.1gCarbohydrates: 6.3g Dietary Fiber: 4g Sugar: 0.1g Protein: 3g

Cheeseburger Chaffle

Servings: 2
Cooking Time: 1
5 Minutes

Ingredients:

- 1 lb. ground beef
- 1 onion, minced
- 1 tsp. parsley, chopped
- 1 egg, beaten
- Salt and pepper to taste
- 1 tablespoon olive oil
- 4 basic chaffles
- 2 lettuce leaves
- 2 cheese slices
- 1 tablespoon dill pickles
- Ketchup
- Mayonnaise

Directions:

1. In a large bowl, combine the ground beef, onion, parsley, egg, salt and pepper.
2. Mix well.
3. Form 2 thick patties.
4. Add olive oil to the pan.
5. Place the pan over medium heat.
6. Cook the patty for 3 to 5 minutes per side or until fully cooked.
7. Place the patty on top of each chaffle.
8. Top with lettuce, cheese and pickles.
9. Squirt ketchup and mayo over the patty and veggies.
10.   Top with another chaffle.

Nutrition:

Calories 325 Total Fat 16.3g Saturated Fat 6.5g
Cholesterol 157mg Sodium 208mg Total Carbohydrate
3g Dietary Fiber 0.7g Total Sugars 1.4g Protein 39.6g
Potassium 532mg

Buffalo Hummus Beef Chaffles

Servings: 4

Cooking Time:

32 Minutes

Ingredients:

- 2 eggs
- 1 cup + ¼ cup finely grated cheddar cheese, divided
- 2 chopped fresh scallions
- Salt and freshly ground black pepper to taste
- 2 chicken breasts, cooked and diced
- ¼ cup buffalo sauce
- 3 tbsp low-carb hummus
- 2 celery stalks, chopped
- ¼ cup crumbled blue cheese for topping

Directions:

1. Preheat the waffle iron.
2. In a medium bowl, mix the eggs, 1 cup of the cheddar cheese, scallions, salt, and black pepper,
3. Open the iron and add a quarter of the mixture. Close and cook until crispy, 7 minutes.
4. Transfer the chaffle to a plate and make 3 more chaffles in the same manner.
5. Preheat the oven to 400 F and line a baking sheet with parchment paper. Set aside.
6. Cut the chaffles into quarters and arrange on the baking sheet.
7. In a medium bowl, mix the chicken with the buffalo sauce, hummus, and celery.

8. Spoon the chicken mixture onto each quarter of chaffles and top with the remaining cheddar cheese.
9. Place the baking sheet in the oven and bake until the cheese melts, 4 minutes.
10.   Remove from the oven and top with the blue cheese.
11.   Serve afterward.

Nutrition:

Calories 552 Fats 28.37g Carbs 6.97g Net Carbs 6.07g Protein 59.8g

Basic Mozzarella Chaffles

Servings: 2
Cooking Time:
6 Minutes

Ingredients:

- 1 large organic egg, beaten
- ½ cup Mozzarella cheese, shredded finely

Directions:

1. Preheat a mini waffle iron and then grease it.
2. In a small bowl, place the egg and Mozzarella cheese and stir to combine.
3. Place half of the mixture into preheated waffle iron and cook for about 2-minutes or until golden brown.
4. Repeat with the remaining mixture.
5. Serve warm.

Nutrition:

Calories: 5 Net Carb: 0.4g Fat: 3.7g Saturated Fat: 1.5g Carbohydrates: 0.4g Dietary Fiber: 0g Sugar: 0.2g Protein: 5.2g

Brie And Blackberry Chaffles

Servings: 4

Cooking Time:

36 Minutes

Ingredients:

- For the chaffles:
- 2 eggs, beaten
- 1 cup finely grated mozzarella cheese
- For the topping:
- 1 ½ cups blackberries
- 1 lemon, 1 tsp zest and 2 tbsp juice
- 1 tbsp erythritol
- 4 slices Brie cheese

Directions:

1. For the chaffles:
2. Preheat the waffle iron.
3. Meanwhile, in a medium bowl, mix the eggs and mozzarella cheese.
4. Open the iron, pour in a quarter of the mixture, cover, and cook until crispy, 7 minutes.
5. Remove the chaffle onto a plate and make 3 more with the remaining batter.
6. Plate and set aside.
7. For the topping:
8. In a medium pot, add the blackberries, lemon zest, lemon juice, and erythritol. Cook until the blackberries break and the sauce thickens, 5 minutes. Turn the heat off.
9. Arrange the chaffles on the baking sheet and place two Brie cheese slices on each. Top with

blackberry mixture and transfer the baking sheet to the oven.

10.   Bake until the cheese melts, 2 to 3 minutes.

11.   Remove from the oven, allow cooling and serve afterward.

Nutrition:

Calories 576 Fats 42.22 g Carbs 7.07 g Net Carbs 3.67 g Protein 42.35 g

Turkey Chaffle Burger

Servings: 2

Cooking Time:

10 Minutes

Ingredients:

- 2 cups ground turkey
- Salt and pepper to taste
- 1 tablespoon olive oil
- 4 garlic chaffles
- 1 cup Romaine lettuce, chopped
- 1 tomato, sliced
- Mayonnaise
- Ketchup

Directions:

1. Combine ground turkey, salt and pepper.
2. Form thick burger patties.
3. Add the olive oil to a pan over medium heat.
4. Cook the turkey burger until fully cooked on both sides.
5. Spread mayo on the chaffle.
6. Top with the turkey burger, lettuce and tomato.
7. Squirt ketchup on top before topping with another chaffle.

Nutrition:

Calories 555 Total Fat 21.5 g Saturated Fat 3.5 g
Cholesterol 117 mg Sodium 654 mg Total Carbohydrate
4.1 g Dietary Fiber 2.5 g Protein 31.7 g Total Sugars 1
g

Double Choco Chaffle

Servings: 2

Cooking Time:

10 Minutes

Ingredients:

- 1 egg
- 2 teaspoons coconut flour
- 2 tablespoons sweetener
- 1 tablespoon cocoa powder
- ¼ teaspoon baking powder
- 1 oz. cream cheese
- ½ teaspoon vanilla
- 1 tablespoon sugar-free chocolate chips

Directions:

1. Put all the ingredients in a large bowl.
2. Mix well.
3. Pour half of the mixture into the waffle maker.
4. Seal the device.
5. Cook for 4 minutes.
6. Uncover and transfer to a plate to cool.
7. Repeat the procedure to make the second chaffle.

Nutrition:

Calories 171 Total Fat 10.7g Saturated Fat 5.3g
Cholesterol 97 mg Sodium 106 mg Potassium 179 mg

Total Carbohydrate 3 g Dietary Fiber 4 Protein 5.8 g
Total Sugars 0.4 g

Guacamole Chaffle Bites

Servings: 2

Cooking Time:

14 Minutes

Ingredients:

- 1 large turnip, cooked and mashed
- 2 bacon slices, cooked and finely chopped
- ½ cup finely grated Monterey Jack cheese
- 1 egg, beaten
- 1 cup guacamole for topping

Directions:

1. Preheat the waffle iron.
2. Mix all the ingredients except for the guacamole in a medium bowl.
3. Open the iron and add half of the mixture. Close and cook for 4 minutes. Open the lid, flip the chaffle and cook further until golden brown and crispy, minutes.
4. Remove the chaffle onto a plate and make another in the same manner.
5. Cut each chaffle into wedges, top with the guacamole and serve afterward.

Nutrition:

Calories 311 Fats 22.52 g Carbs 8.29g Net Carbs 5.79 g Protein 13 g

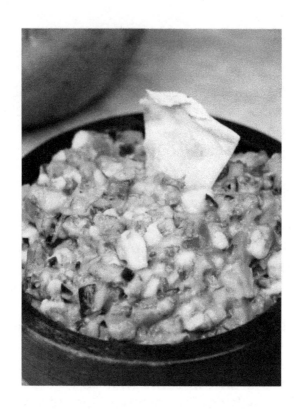

Mayonnaise & Cream Cheese Chaffles

Servings: 4
Cooking Time:
20 Minutes

Ingredients:

- 4 organic eggs large
- 4 tablespoons mayonnaise
- 1 tablespoon almond flour
- 2 tablespoons cream cheese, cut into small cubes

Directions:

1. Preheat a waffle iron and then grease it.
2. In a bowl, place the eggs, mayonnaise and almond flour and with a hand mixer, mix until smooth.
3. Place about ¼ of the mixture into preheated waffle iron.
4. Place about ¼ of the cream cheese cubes on top of the mixture evenly and cook for about 5 minutes or until golden brown.
5. Repeat with the remaining mixture and cream cheese cubes.
6. Serve warm.

Nutrition:

Calories: 190 Net Carb: 0.6g Fat: 17 g Saturated Fat: 4.2 g Carbohydrates: 0.8 g Dietary Fiber: 0.2 g Sugar: 0.5 g Protein: 6.7 g

Blue Cheese Chaffle Bites

Servings: 2

Cooking Time:

14 Minutes

Ingredients:

- 1 egg, beaten
- ½ cup finely grated Parmesan cheese
- ¼ cup crumbled blue cheese
- 1 tsp erythritol

Directions:

1. Preheat the waffle iron.
2. Mix all the ingredients in a bowl.
3. Open the iron and add half of the mixture. Close and cook until crispy, 7 minutes.
4. Remove the chaffle onto a plate and make another with the remaining mixture.
5. Cut each chaffle into wedges and serve afterward.

Nutrition:

Calories: 19 Net Carbs: 4.03 g Protein 13.48g

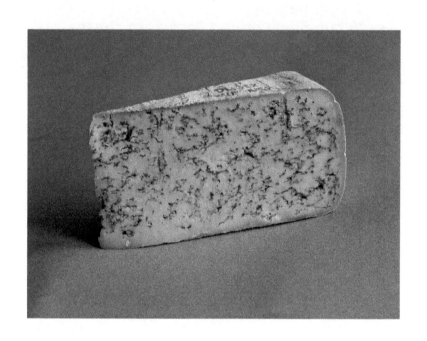

Raspberries Chaffles

Servings: 2

Cooking Time:

5 Minutes

Ingredients:

- 1 egg
- 1/2 cup mozzarella cheese, shredded
- 1 tbsp. almond flour
- 1/4 cup raspberry puree
- 1 tbsp. coconut flour for topping

Directions:

1. Preheat your waffle makerin line with the manufacturer's instructions.
2. Grease your waffle maker with cooking spray.
3. Mix together egg, almond flour, and raspberry purée.
4. Add cheese and mix until well combined.
5. Pour batter intothe waffle maker.
6. Close the lid.
7. Cook for about 3-4 minutesutes or until waffles are cooked and not soggy.
8. Once cooked, remove from the maker.
9. Sprinkle coconut flour on top and enjoy!

Nutrition:

Protein: 26% 60 kcal Fat: 63% 145 kcal Carbohydrates: 11% 25 kcal

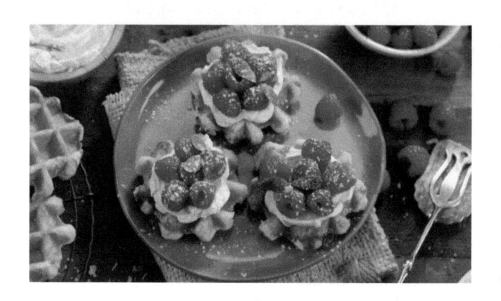

Simple Chaffle Toast

Servings:2
Cooking Time:
5 Minutes

Ingredients:

- 1 large egg
- 1/2 cup shredded cheddar cheese
- FOR TOPPING
- 1 egg
- 3-4 spinach leaves
- ¼ cup boil and shredded chicken

Directions:

1. Preheat your square waffle maker on medium-high heat.
2. Mix together egg and cheese in a bowl and make two chaffles in a chaffle maker
3. Once chaffle are cooked, carefully remove them from the maker.
4. Serve with spinach, boiled chicken, and fried egg.
5. Serve hot and enjoy!

Nutrition:

Protein: 39% 99 kcal Fat: % 153 kcal Carbohydrates: 1% 3 kcal

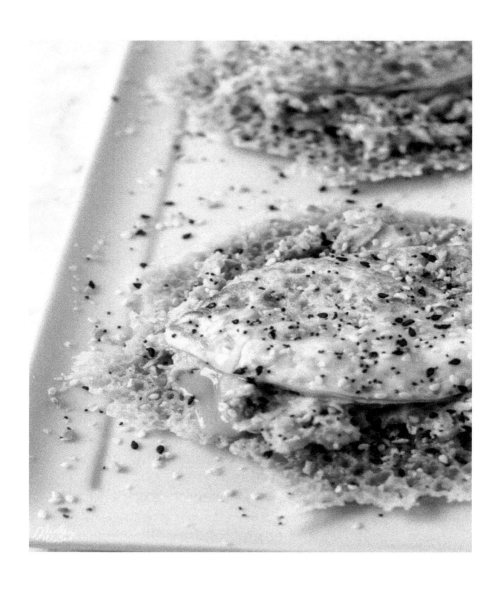

Savory Beef Chaffle

Servings: 2

Cooking Time:

15 Minutes

Ingredients:

- 1 teaspoon olive oil
- 2 cups ground beef
- Garlic salt to taste
- 1 red bell pepper, sliced into strips
- 1 green bell pepper, sliced into strips
- 1 onion, minced
- 1 bay leaf
- 2 garlic chaffles
- Butter

Directions:

1. Put your pan over medium heat.
2. Add the olive oil and cook ground beef until brown.
3. Season with garlic salt and add bay leaf.
4. Drain the fat, transfer to a plate and set aside.
5. Discard the bay leaf.
6. In the same pan, cook the onion and bell peppers for 2 minutes.
7. Put the beef back to the pan.
8. Heat for 1 minute.
9. Spread butter on top of the chaffle.
10. Add the ground beef and veggies.
11. Roll or fold the chaffle.

Nutrition:

Calories 220 Total Fat 17.8 g Saturated Fat 8 g
Cholesterol 76 mg Sodium 60 mg Total Carbohydrate 3
g Dietary Fiber 2 g Total Sugars 5.4 g Protein 27.1 g
Potassium 537 mg

Chaffles With Almond Flour

Servings:4

Cooking Time:

5 Minutes

Ingredients:

- 2 large eggs
- 1/4 cup almond flour
- 3/4 tsp baking powder
- 1 cup cheddar cheese, shredded
- Cooking spray

Directions:

1. Switch on your waffle maker and grease with cooking spray.
2. Beat eggs with almond flour and baking powder in a mixing bowl.
3. Once the eggs and cheese are mixed together, add in cheese and mix again.
4. Pour 1/cup of the batter in the dash mini waffle maker and close the lid.
5. Cook chaffles for about 2-3 minutes until crispy and cooked
6. Repeat with the remaining batter
7. Carefully transfer the chafflesto plate.
8. Serve with almonds and enjoy!

Nutrition:

Protein: 23% 52 kcal Fat: 72% 15kcal Carbohydrates: 5% 11 kcal

Nutter Butter Chaffles

Servings: 2
Cooking Time:
14 Minutes

Ingredients:

- For the chaffles:
- 2 tbsp sugar-free peanut butter powder
- 2 tbsp maple (sugar-free) syrup
- 1 egg, beaten
- ¼ cup finely grated mozzarella cheese
- ¼ tsp baking powder
- ¼ tsp almond butter
- ¼ tsp peanut butter extract
- 1 tbsp softened cream cheese
- For the frosting:
- ½ cup almond flour
- 1 cup peanut butter
- 3 tbsp almond milk
- ½ tsp vanilla extract
- ½ cup maple (sugar-free) syrup

Directions:

1. Preheat the waffle iron.
2. Meanwhile, in a medium bowl, mix all the ingredients until smooth.
3. Open the iron and pour in half of the mixture.
4. Close the iron and cook until crispy, 6 to 7 minutes.
5. Remove the chaffle onto a plate and set aside.
6. Make a second chaffle with the remaining batter.
7. While the chaffles cool, make the frosting.

8. Pour the almond flour in a medium saucepan and stir-fry over medium heat until golden.
9. Transfer the almond flour to a blender and top with the remaining frosting ingredients. Process until smooth.
10. Spread the frosting on the chaffles and serve afterward.

Nutrition:

Calories 239 Fats 15.48 g Carbs 17.42 g Net Carbs 15.92 g Protein 7.52 g

Hot Dog Chaffles

Servings: 2

Cooking Time:

14 Minutes

Ingredients:

- 1 egg, beaten
- 1 cup finely grated cheddar cheese
- 2 hot dog sausages, cooked
- Mustard dressing for topping
- 8 pickle slices

Directions:

1. Preheat the waffle iron.
2. In a medium bowl, mix the egg and cheddar cheese.
3. Open the iron and add half of the mixture. Close and cook until crispy, 7 minutes.
4. Transfer the chaffle to a plate and make a second chaffle in the same manner.
5. To serve, top each chaffle with a sausage, swirl the mustard dressing on top, and then divide the pickle slices on top.
6. Enjoy!

Nutrition:

Calories 231Fats 18.29gCarbs 2.8gNet Carbs 2.6gProtein 13.39g

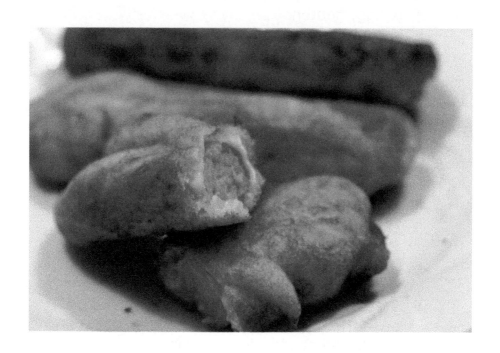

Keto Reuben Chaffles

Servings: 4

Cooking Time:

28 Minutes

Ingredients:

- For the chaffles:
- 2 eggs, beaten
- 1 cup finely grated Swiss cheese
- 2 tsp caraway seeds
- 1/8 tsp salt
- ½ tsp baking powder
- For the sauce:
- 2 tbsp sugar-free ketchup
- 3 tbsp mayonnaise
- 1 tbsp dill relish
- 1 tsp hot sauce
- For the filling:
- 6 oz pastrami
- 2 Swiss cheese slices
- ¼ cup pickled radishes

Directions:

1. For the chaffles:
2. Preheat the waffle iron.
3. In a medium bowl, mix the eggs, Swiss cheese, caraway seeds, salt, and baking powder.
4. Open the iron and add a quarter of the mixture. Close and cook until crispy, 7 minutes.
5. Transfer the chaffle to a plate and make 3 more chaffles in the same manner.

6. For the sauce:
7. In another bowl, mix the ketchup, mayonnaise, dill relish, and hot sauce.
8. To assemble:
9. Divide on two chaffles; the sauce, the pastrami, Swiss cheese slices, and pickled radishes.
10. Cover with the other chaffles, divide the sandwich in halves and serve.

Nutrition:

Calories 316 Fats 21.78 g Carbs 6.52 g Net Carbs 5.42 g Protein 23.56 g

Carrot Chaffle Cake

Servings: 6

Cooking Time:

24 Minutes

Ingredients:

- 1 egg, beaten
- 2 tablespoons melted butter
- ½ cup carrot, shredded
- ¾ cup almond flour
- 1 teaspoon baking powder
- 2 tablespoons heavy whipping cream
- 2 tablespoons sweetener
- 1 tablespoon walnuts, chopped
- 1 teaspoon pumpkin spice
- 2 teaspoons cinnamon

Directions:

1. Preheat your waffle maker.
2. In a large bowl, combine all the ingredients.
3. Pour some of the mixture into the waffle maker.
4. Close and cook for minutes.
5. Repeat steps until all the remaining batter has been used.

Nutrition:

Calories 294 Total Fat 27 g Saturated Fat 12 g
Cholesterol 133 mg Sodium 144 mg Potassium 421 mg

Total Carbohydrate 11.6 g Dietary Fiber 4.5 g Protein 6.8 g Total Sugars 1.7 g

Colby Jack Slices Chaffles

Servings: 1
Cooking Time:
6 Minutes

Ingredients:

- 2 ounces Colby Jack cheese, cut into thin triangle slices
- 1 large organic egg, beaten

Directions:

1. Preheat a waffle iron and then grease it.
2. Arrange 1 thin layer of cheese slices in the bottom of preheated waffle iron.
3. Place the beaten egg on top of the cheese.
4. Now, arrange another layer of cheese slices on top to cover evenly.
5. Cook for about 6 minutes or until golden brown.
6. Serve warm.

Nutrition:

Calories: 292 Net Carb: 2.4 g Fat: 23 g Saturated Fat: 13.6 g Carbohydrates: 2.4 g Dietary Fiber: 0 g Sugar: 0.4 g Protein: 18.3 g

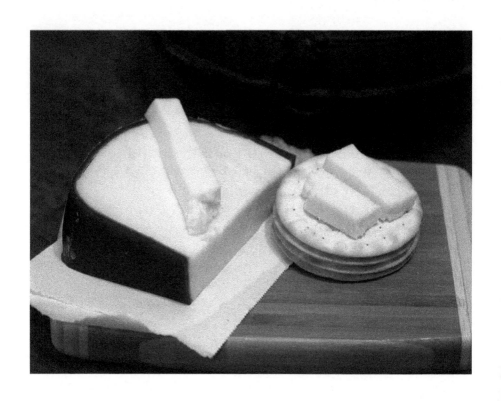

Egg & Chives Chaffle Sandwich Roll

Servings: 2

Cooking Time:

0 Minute

Ingredients:

- 2 tablespoons mayonnaise
- 1 hard-boiled egg, chopped
- 1 tablespoon chives, chopped
- 2 basic chaffles

Directions:

1. In a bowl, mix the mayo, egg and chives.
2. Spread the mixture on top of the chaffles.
3. Roll the chaffle.

Nutrition:

Calories 258 Total Fat 12g Saturated Fat 2.8 g
Cholesterol 171 mg Sodium 271 mg Potassium 71mg
Total Carbohydrate 7.5 g Dietary Fiber 0.1 g Protein 5.9
g Total Sugars 2.3 g

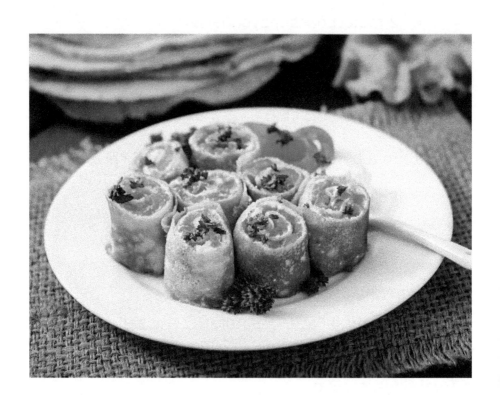

Basic Chaffles Recipe For Sandwiches

Servings:2

Cooking Time:

5 Minutes

Ingredients:

- 1/2 cup mozzarella cheese, shredded
- 1 large egg
- 2 tbsps.almond flour
- 1/2 tsp psyllium husk powder
- 1/4 tsp baking powder

Directions:

1. Grease your Belgian waffle maker with cooking spray.
2. Beat the egg with a fork; once the egg is beaten, add almond flour, husk powder, and baking powder.
3. Add cheesetothe egg mixture and mix until combined.
4. Pour batter in the center of Belgian waffle and close the lid.
5. Cook chaffles for about 2-3 minutesutes until well cooked.
6. Carefully transfer the chaffles to plate.
7. The chaffles are perfect for a sandwich base.

Nutrition:

Protein: 29% 60 kcal Fat: 63% 132 kcal Carbohydrates: 18 kcal

Cereal Chaffle Cake

Servings: 2

Cooking Time:

8 Minutes

Ingredients:

- 1 egg
- 2 tablespoons almond flour
- ½ teaspoon coconut flour
- 1 tablespoon melted butter
- 1 tablespoon cream cheese
- 1 tablespoon plain cereal, crushed
- ¼ teaspoon vanilla extract
- ¼ teaspoon baking powder
- 1 tablespoon sweetener
- 1/8 teaspoon xanthan gum

Directions:

1. Plug in your waffle maker to preheat.
2. Add all the ingredients in a large bowl.
3. Mix until well blended.
4. Let the batter rest for 2 minutes before cooking.
5. Pour half of the mixture into the waffle maker.
6. Seal and cook for 4 minutes.
7. Make the next chaffle using the same steps.

Nutrition:

Calories 154 Total Fat 21.2 g Saturated Fat 10 g
Cholesterol 113.3 mg Sodium 96.9 mg Potassium 453
mg Total Carbohydrate 5.9 g Dietary Fiber 1.7 g Protein
4.6 g Total Sugars 2.7 g

Okonomiyaki Chaffles

Servings: 4

Cooking Time:

28 Minutes

Ingredients:

- For the chaffles:
- 2 eggs, beaten
- 1 cup finely grated mozzarella cheese
- ½ tsp baking powder
- ¼ cup shredded radishes
- For the sauce:
- 2 tsp coconut aminos
- 2 tbsp sugar-free ketchup
- 1 tbsp sugar-free maple syrup
- 2 tsp Worcestershire sauce
- For the topping:
- 1 tbsp mayonnaise
- 2 tbsp chopped fresh scallions
- 2 tbsp bonito flakes
- 1 tsp dried seaweed powder
- 1 tbsp pickled ginger

Directions:

1. For the chaffles:
2. Preheat the waffle iron.
3. In a medium bowl, mix the eggs, mozzarella cheese, baking powder, and radishes.
4. Open the iron and add a quarter of the mixture. Close and cook until crispy, 7 minutes.
5. Transfer the chaffle to a plate and make a 3 more chaffles in the same manner.

6. For the sauce:
7. Combine the coconut aminos, ketchup, maple syrup, and Worcestershire sauce in a medium bowl and mix well.
8. For the topping:
9. In another mixing bowl, mix the mayonnaise, scallions, bonito flakes, seaweed powder, and ginger
10.   To Servings:
11.   Arrange the chaffles on four different plates and swirl the sauce on top. Spread the topping on the chaffles and serve afterward.

Nutrition:

Calories 90 Fats 3.32 g Carbs 2.97g Net Carbs 2.17 g Protein 09 g

Bacon & Chicken Ranch Chaffle

Servings: 2
Cooking Time:
8 Minutes

Ingredients:

- 1 egg
- ¼ cup chicken cubes, cooked
- 1 slice bacon, cooked and chopped
- ¼ cup cheddar cheese, shredded
- 1 teaspoon ranch dressing powder

Directions:

1. Preheat your waffle maker.
2. In a bowl, mix all the ingredients.
3. Add half of the mixture to your waffle maker.
4. Cover and cook for minutes.
5. Make the second chaffle using the same steps.

Nutrition:

Calories 200Total Fat 14 g Saturated Fat g Cholesterol 129 mg Sodium 463 mg Potassium 130 mgTotal Carbohydrate 2 g Dietary Fiber 1 g Protein 16 g Total Sugars 1 g

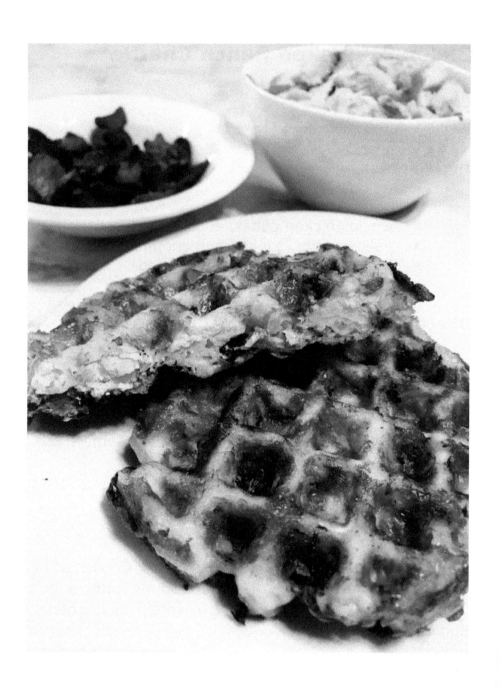

Keto Cocoa Chaffles

Servings: 2
Cooking Time:
5 Minutes

Ingredients:

- 1 large egg
- 1/2 cup shredded cheddar cheese
- 1 tbsp. cocoa powder
- 2 tbsps. almond flour

Directions:

1. Preheat your round waffle maker on medium-high heat.
2. Mix together egg, cheese, almond flour, cocoa powder and vanilla in a small mixing bowl.
3. Pour chaffles mixture into the center of the waffle iron.
4. Close the waffle maker and let cook for 3-5 minutesutes or until waffle is golden brown and set.
5. Carefully remove chaffles from the waffle maker.
6. Serve hot and enjoy!

Nutrition:

Protein: 20% 49 kcal Fat: % 183 kcal Carbohydrates: 7% 17 kcal

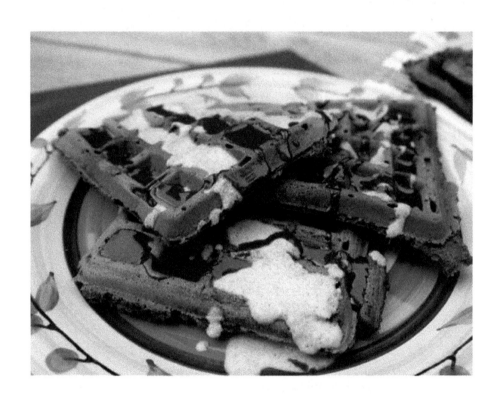

Barbecue Chaffle

Servings: 2

Cooking Time:

8 Minutes

Ingredients:

- 1 egg, beaten
- ½ cup cheddar cheese, shredded
- ½ teaspoon barbecue sauce
- ¼ teaspoon baking powder

Directions:

1. Plug in your waffle maker to preheat.
2. Mix all the ingredients in a bowl.
3. Pour half of the mixture to your waffle maker.
4. Cover and cook for minutes.
5. Repeat the same steps for the next barbecue chaffle.

Nutrition:

Calories 295 Total Fat 23 g Saturated Fat 13 g
Cholesterol 223 mg Sodium 414 mg Potassium 179 mg
Total Carbohydrate 2 g Dietary Fiber 1 g Protein 20 g
Total Sugars 1 g

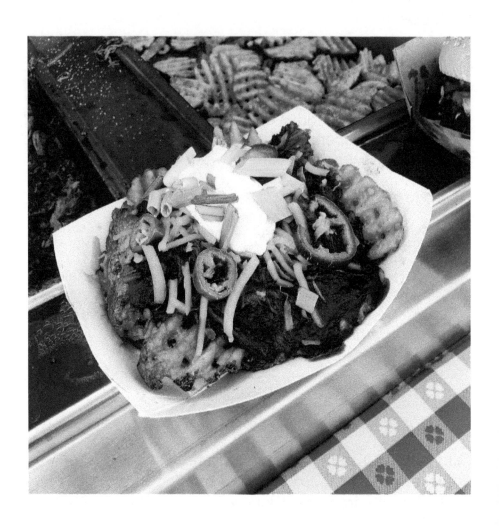

Chicken And Chaffle Nachos

Servings: 4

Cooking Time:

33 Minutes

Ingredients:

- For the chaffles:
- 2 eggs, beaten
- 1 cup finely grated Mexican cheese blend
- For the chicken-cheese topping:
- 2 tbsp butter
- 1 tbsp almond flour
- ¼ cup unsweetened almond milk
- 1 cup finely grated cheddar cheese + more to garnish
- 3 bacon slices, cooked and chopped
- 2 cups cooked and diced chicken breasts
- 2 tbsp hot sauce
- 2 tbsp chopped fresh scallions

Directions:

1. For the chaffles:
2. Preheat the waffle iron.
3. In a medium bowl, mix the eggs and Mexican cheese blend.
4. Open the iron and add a quarter of the mixture. Close and cook until crispy, 7 minutes.
5. Transfer the chaffle to a plate and make 3 more chaffles in the same manner.
6. Place the chaffles on serving plates and set aside for serving.
7. For the chicken-cheese topping:

8. Melt the butter in a large skillet and mix in the almond flour until brown, 1 minute.
9. Pour the almond milk and whisk until well combined. Simmer until thickened, 2 minutes.
10.   Stir in the cheese to melt, 2 minutes and then mix in the bacon, chicken, and hot sauce.
11.   Spoon the mixture onto the chaffles and top with some more cheddar cheese.
12.   Garnish with the scallions and serve immediately.

Nutrition:

Calories 524 Fats 37.51 g Carbs 3.55g Net Carbs 3.25 g Protein 41.86 g

Ham, Cheese & Tomato Chaffle Sandwich

Servings: 2

Cooking Time:

10 Minutes

Ingredients:

- 1 teaspoon olive oil
- 2 slices ham
- 4 basic chaffles
- 1 tablespoon mayonnaise
- 2 slices Provolone cheese
- 1 tomato, sliced

Directions:

1. Add the olive oil to a pan over medium heat.
2. Cook the ham for 1 minute per side.
3. Spread the chaffles with mayonnaise.
4. Top with the ham, cheese and tomatoes.
5. Top with another chaffle to make a sandwich.

Nutrition:

Calories 198 Total Fat 14.7 g Saturated Fat 3 g Cholesterol 37 mg Sodium 664 mg Total Carbohydrate 4.6g Dietary Fiber 0.7 g Total Sugars 1.5 g Protein 12.2 g Potassium 193 mg

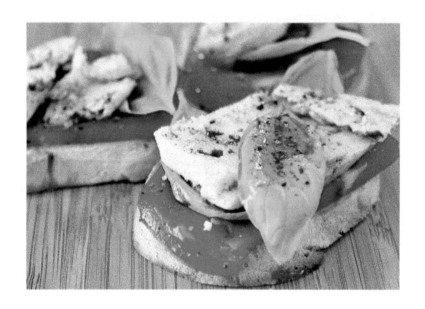

Basic Keto Chaffles

Servings: 2

Cooking Time:

5 Minutes

Ingredients:

- 1 egg
- ½ cup shredded Cheddar cheese

Directions:

1. Turn on waffle maker to heat and oil it with cooking spray.
2. Whisk egg in a bowl until well beaten.
3. Add cheese to the egg and stir well to combine.
4. Pour ½ batter into the waffle maker and close the top. Cook for 3-5 minutes.
5. Transfer chaffle to a plate and set aside for 2-3 minutes to crisp up.
6. Repeat for remaining batter.

Nutrition:

Carbs: 1 g ;Fat: 12 g ;Protein: 9 g ;Calories: 150

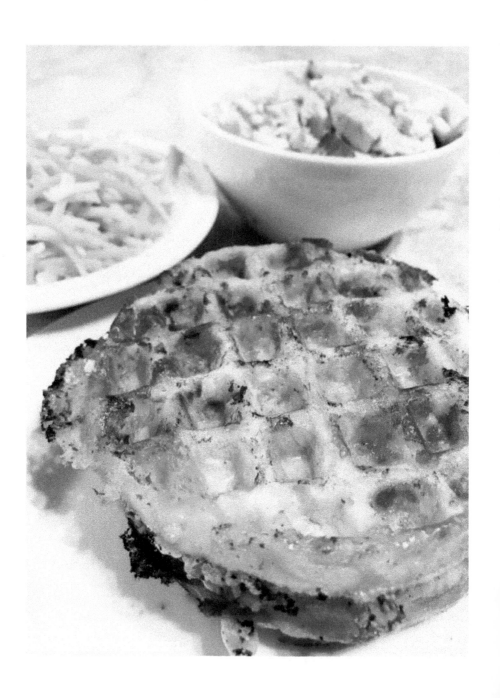

Red Velvet Chaffles

Servings: 2

Cooking Time:

8 Minutes

Ingredients:

- 2 tablespoons cacao powder
- 2 tablespoons erythritol
- 1 organic egg, beaten
- 2 drops super red food coloring
- ¼ teaspoon organic baking powder
- 1 tablespoon heavy whipping cream

Directions:

1. Preheat a mini waffle iron and then grease it.
2. In a medium bowl, put all ingredients and with a fork, mix until well combined.
3. Place half of the mixture into preheated waffle iron and cook for about 4 minutes.
4. Repeat with the remaining mixture.
5. Serve warm.

Nutrition:

Calories 70 Net Carbs 1.7 g Total Fat g Saturated Fat 3 g Cholesterol 92 mg Sodium 34 mg Total Carbs 3.2 g Fiber 1.5 g Sugar 0.2 g Protein 3.9 g

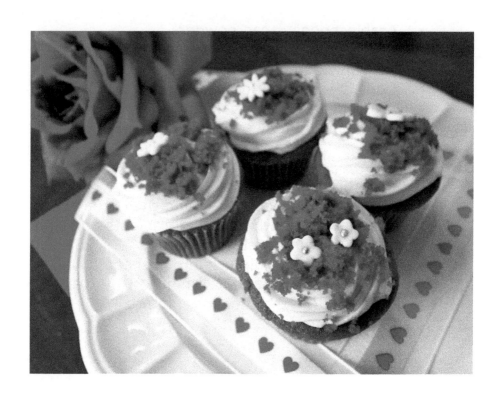

Mayonnaise Chaffles

Servings: 2

Cooking Time:

10 Minutes

Ingredients:

- 1 large organic egg, beaten1 tablespoon mayonnaise
- 2 tablespoons almond flour
- 1/8 teaspoon organic baking powder
- 1 teaspoon water2–4 drops liquid stevia

Directions:

1. Preheat a mini waffle iron and then grease it.
2. In a medium bowl, put all ingredients and with a fork, mix until well combined. Place half of the mixture into preheated waffle iron and cook for about 4–5 minutes.
3. Repeat with the remaining mixture.
4. Serve warm.

Nutrition:

Calories 110 Net Carbs 2.6 g Total Fat 8.7 g Saturated Fat 1.4 g Cholesterol 9mg Sodium 88 g Total Carbs 3.4 g Fiber 0.8 g Sugar 0.9 g Protein 3.2 g

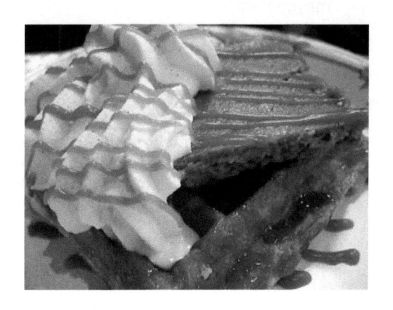

Chocolate Peanut Butter Chaffle

Servings: 2

Cooking Time:

10 Minutes

Ingredients:

- ½ cup shredded mozzarella cheese
- 1 Tbsp cocoa powder
- 2 Tbsp powdered sweetener
- 2 Tbsp peanut butter
- ½ tsp vanilla
- 1 egg
- 2 Tbsp crushed peanuts
- 2 Tbsp whipped cream
- ¼ cup sugar-free chocolate syrup

Directions:

1. Combine mozzarella, egg, vanilla, peanut butter, cocoa powder, and sweetener in a bowl.
2. Add in peanuts and mix well.
3. Turn on waffle maker and oil it with cooking spray.
4. Pour one half of the batter into waffle maker and cook for minutes, then transfer to a plate.
5. Top with whipped cream, peanuts, and sugar-free chocolate syrup.

Nutrition:

Carbs: g ;Fat: 17 g ;Protein: 15 g ;Calories: 236

Lemon Curd Chaffles

Servings: 1

Cooking Time:

5 Minutes

Ingredients:

- 3 large eggs
- 4 oz cream cheese, softened
- 1 Tbsp low carb sweetener
- 1 tsp vanilla extract
- ¾ cup mozzarella cheese, shredded
- 3 Tbsp coconut flour
- 1 tsp baking powder
- ⅓ tsp salt
- For the lemon curd:
- ½-1 cup water
- 5 egg yolks
- ½ cup lemon juice
- ½ cup powdered sweetener
- 2 Tbsp fresh lemon zest
- 1 tsp vanilla extract
- Pinch of salt
- 8 Tbsp cold butter, cubed

Directions:

1. Pour water into a saucepan and heat over medium until it reaches a soft boil. Start with ½ cup and add more if needed.
2. Whisk yolks, lemon juice, lemon zest, powdered sweetener, vanilla, and salt in a medium heat-proof bowl. Leave to set for 5-6 minutes.
3. Place bowl onto saucepan and heat. The bowl shouldn't be touching water.

4. Whisk mixture for 8-10 minutes, or until it begins to thicken.
5. Add butter cubes and whisk for 7 minutes, until it thickens.
6. When it lightly coats the back of a spoon, remove from heat.
7. Refrigerate until cool, allowing it to continue thickening.
8. Turn on waffle maker to heat and oil it with cooking spray.
9. Add baking powder, coconut flour, and salt in a small bowl. Mix well and set aside.
10. Add eggs, cream cheese, sweetener, and vanilla in a separate bowl. Using a hand beater, beat until frothy.
11. Add mozzarella to egg mixture and beat again.
12. Add dry ingredients and mix until well-combined.
13. Add batter to waffle maker and cook for 3-4 minutes.
14. Transfer to a plate and top with lemon curd before serving.

Nutrition:

Carbs: 6 g; Fat: 24 g ; Protein: g Calories –302

Walnut Pumpkin Chaffles

Servings: 2

Cooking Time:

10 Minutes

Ingredients:

- 1 organic egg, beaten
- ½ cup Mozzarella cheese, shredded
- 2 tablespoons almond flour
- 1 tablespoon sugar-free pumpkin puree
- 1 teaspoon Erythritol
- ¼ teaspoon ground cinnamon
- 2 tablespoons walnuts, toasted and chopped

Directions:

1. Preheat a mini waffle iron and then grease it.
2. In a bowl, place all ingredients except walnuts and beat until well combined.
3. Fold in the walnuts.
4. Place half of the mixture into preheated waffle iron and cook for about 5 minutes or until golden brown.
5. Repeat with the remaining mixture.
6. Serve warm.

Nutrition:

Calories: 148 Net Carb: 1.6g Fat: 11.8 g Saturated Fat: 2 g Carbohydrates: 3.3 g Dietary Fiber: 1 Sugar: 0.8 g Protein: 6.7 g

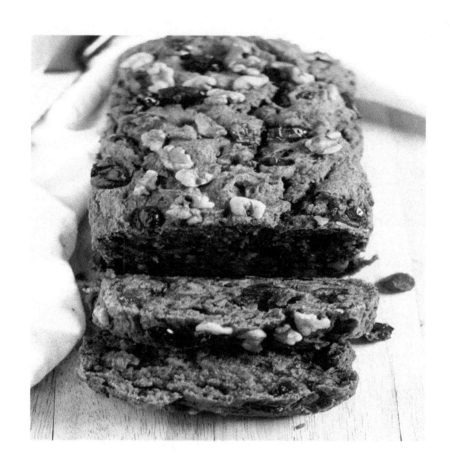

Protein Mozzarella Chaffles

Servings: 4

Cooking Time:

20 Minutes

Ingredients:

- ½ scoop unsweetened protein powder
- 2 large organic eggs
- ½ cup Mozzarella cheese, shredded
- 1 tablespoon Erythritol
- ¼ teaspoon organic vanilla extract

Directions:

1. Preheat a mini waffle iron and then grease it.
2. In a medium bowl, place all ingredients and with a fork, mix until well combined.
3. Place ¼ of the mixture into preheated waffle iron and cook for about 4-5 minutes or until golden brown.
4. Repeat with the remaining mixture.
5. Serve warm.

Nutrition:

Calories: Net Carb: 0.4 g Fat: 3.3 g Saturated Fat: 1.2 g Carbohydrates: 0.4 g Dietary Fiber: 0 g Sugar: 0.2 g Protein: 7.3 g

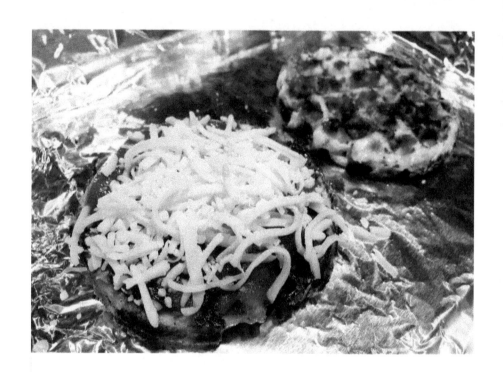

Chocolate Chips Peanut Butter Chaffles

Servings: 2

Cooking Time:

8 Minutes

Ingredients:

- 1 organic egg, beaten
- ¼ cup Mozzarella cheese, shredded
- 2 tablespoons creamy peanut butter
- 1 tablespoon almond flour
- 1 tablespoon granulated Erythritol
- 1 teaspoon organic vanilla extract
- 1 tablespoon 70% dark chocolate chips

Directions:

1. Preheat a mini waffle iron and then grease it.
2. In a bowl, place all ingredients except chocolate chips and beat until well combined.
3. Gently, fold in the chocolate chips.
4. Place half of the mixture into preheated waffle iron and cook for about minutes or until golden brown.
5. Repeat with the remaining mixture.
6. Serve warm.

Nutrition:

Calories: 214 Net Carb: 4.1 g Fat: 16.8 g Saturated
Fat: 5.4 g Carbohydrates: 6.4 g Dietary Fiber: 2.3 g
Sugar: 2.1 g Protein: 8.8 g

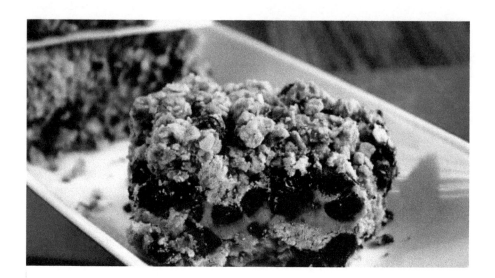

Pumpkin Chaffles

Servings: 2

Cooking Time:

12 Minutes

Ingredients:

- 1 organic egg, beaten
- ½ cup Mozzarella cheese, shredded
- 1½ tablespoon homemade pumpkin puree
- ½ teaspoon Erythritol
- ½ teaspoon organic vanilla extract
- ¼ teaspoon pumpkin pie spice

Directions:

1. Preheat a mini waffle iron and then grease it.
2. In a bowl, place all the ingredients and beat until well combined.
3. Place ¼ of the mixture into preheated waffle iron and cook for about 4-6 minutes or until golden brown.
4. Repeat with the remaining mixture.
5. Serve warm.

Nutrition:

Calories: 59 Net Carb: 1.2 g Fat: 3.5 g Saturated Fat: 1.5 g Carbohydrates: 1 Dietary Fiber: 0.4 g Sugar: 0.7 g Protein: 4.9 g

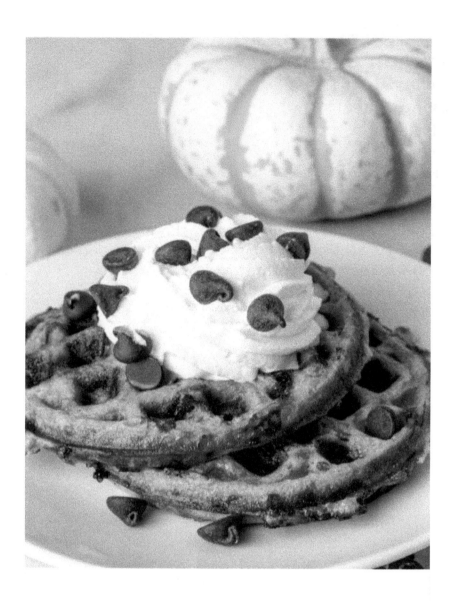

Peanut Butter Chaffles

Servings: 2
Cooking Time:
8 Minutes

Ingredients:

- 1 organic egg, beaten
- ½ cup Mozzarella cheese, shredded
- 3 tablespoons granulated Erythritol
- 2 tablespoons peanut butter

Directions:

1. Preheat a mini waffle iron and then grease it.
2. In a medium bowl, place all ingredients and with a fork, mix until well combined.
3. Place half of the mixture into preheated waffle iron and cook for about 4 minutes or until golden brown.
4. Repeat with the remaining mixture.
5. Serve warm.

Nutrition Info for Servings:

Calories: 145 Net Carb: 2 Fat: 11.5 g Saturated Fat: 3.1 g Carbohydrates: 3.6 g Dietary Fiber: 1 g Sugar: 1.7 g Protein: 8.8 g

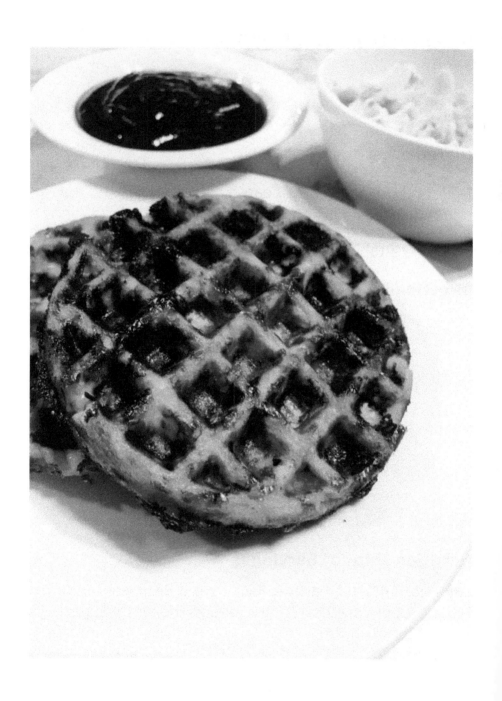

Chocolate Chips Chaffles

Servings: 2

Cooking Time:

8 Minutes

Ingredients:

- 1 large organic egg
- 1 teaspoon coconut flour
- 1 teaspoon Erythritol
- ½ teaspoon organic vanilla extract
- ½ cup Mozzarella cheese, shredded finely
- 2 tablespoons 70% dark chocolate chips

Directions:

1. Preheat a mini waffle iron and then grease it.
2. In a bowl, place the egg, coconut flour, sweetener and vanilla extract and beat until well combined.
3. Add the cheese and stir to combine.
4. Place half of the mixture into preheated waffle iron and top with half of the chocolate chips.
5. Place a little egg mixture over each chocolate chip.
6. Cook for about 3-4 minutes or until golden brown.
7. Repeat with the remaining mixture and chocolate chips.
8. Serve warm.

Nutrition:

Calories: 164 Net Carb: 2 Fat: 11.9 g Saturated Fat:
6.6 g Carbohydrates: 5.4 g Dietary Fiber: 2.5g Sugar:
0.3 g Protein: 7.3 g

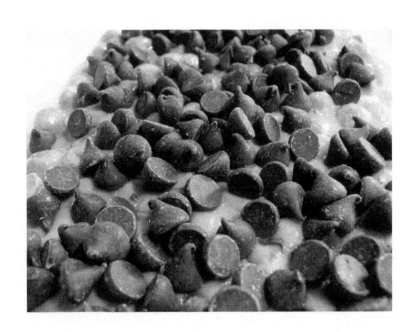

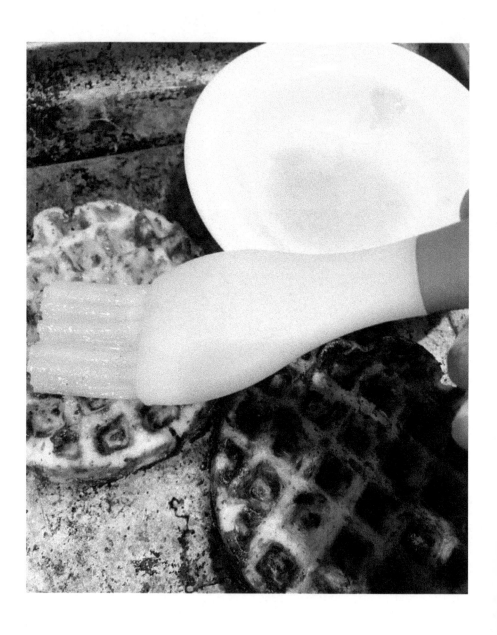

Lightning Source UK Ltd.
Milton Keynes UK
UKHW020800230621
386011UK00006B/66